I0438442

Rev. Carol S. Batey, Ph.D.
Nashville, TN

First published by Carol S. Batey   May 2011

ISBN 978 146 1092 810

Printed in the United States of America
Nashville, Tennessee

This book is printed on acid-free paper.

Before Thought ...

"My voice You shall hear in the morning, O Lord; In the morning I will direct to You, and I will look up." (Psalm 5:3)

If you long to live your life the way it is meant to be lived through "Christ in you, the hope of glory," (Colossians 1:27), then *Developing A Mystic Consciousness* is a must read. It is a most inspired account of God's Grace working in human life.

Carol S. Batey writes with the confidence of experience. She has shown us through her own experience what mysticism truly is: insight into an entirely new world of living. Take your time with this book - assimilate its words, ideas, and courses of action into your heart, soul, mind, and body. You will be moved into a healthier, happier, richer way of living.

This book outlines the necessary steps towards a higher consciousness, including easily followed instructions. You will come to understand how to "let go and let God," and be victorious over the circumstances of your life.

"We have the mind of Christ." (1 Corinthians 2:16)

Your mind has a marvelous ability to adapt, to change, and to create a new life for you. Use it as you are *Developing A Mystic Consciousness.*

Wanda L. Lynch
Licensed First Church Unity Teacher/Counselor
Nashville, TN 37220

About the Author

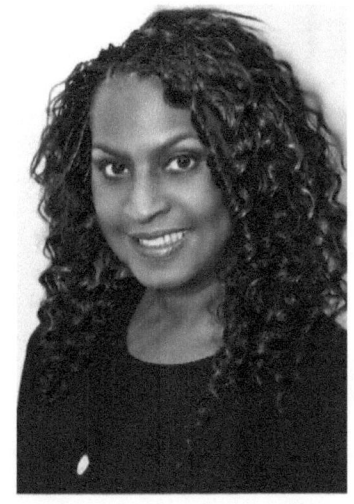

Rev. Carol S. Batey, Ph.D., author of *Parents Are Lifesavers* (Corwin Press 1996), *In Due Season: Destiny's Calling Your Soul* (AuthorHouse 2007), *Poise for the Runway of Your Life* (AuthorHouse 2009), *What's Cooking in Your Soul?* (AuthorHouse 2010), and *Why Aren't You Writing?* (Westry Wingate 2011), is committed to sharing information about how one can improve and renew the purpose of one's soul. Carol provides coaching workshops and seminars for anyone who desires to step into their destiny.

Carol recently earned and received her Doctoral degree in Metaphysics, at the University of Metaphysics at the University of Sedona. Carol has worked as a Parent Involvement Consultant for the Metropolitan Nashville Public Schools in Tennessee. She has received national recognition from educators for her work in parent involvement. During the 1992 school year, she was nominated for the J.C. Penny Golden Rule Award, which is an award to individuals who have performed outstanding service to the local community. Her school won $1,000.00. Over the past seventeen years, Carol has appeared on TV, radio, national Internet radio programs, and newsprint.

Carol was born and raised in Nashville, Tennessee. She is the mother of six adult children, the author of numerous magazine and newspaper articles, and YouTube videos. Carol was educated in the Metropolitan Nashville Public Schools, and has obtained multiple Associate Degrees in business from various schools in Nashville. She is a visual artist and the creator of her own skin care line. The cover of this book is an original painting by Carol and is currently for sale.

At age 51, Carol became a Lifestyle Model for Elite Models in Atlanta, Georgia, managed by Sharon Smith Talent. She has worked in the performing arts on various assignments. Her workshops "*Your Destiny Awaits You*" and "*Hold on to Your Dreams*" are very popular. Attendees receive instruction, which allows them to leave with new knowledge, motivation, and a sense of self-empowerment. Her signature class is "*Why Aren't You Writing?*"

She welcomes your e-mails or personal calls for speaking, coaching, retreats, and workshops for your organization, or yourself.

Contact Carol at:

Email: carol37076@aol.com

Phone: (615) 485-4548

Website: www.artlifestylecoach.com

Blog: www.carolsbatey.blogspot.com

You can also find Carol on Facebook and You Tube.

4

Table of Contents

"When entering the Silence, close the eyes and ears to the without. Go
to [Divine Mind] within [consciousness] and hold the mind steadily
on the word until that word illumines the whole inner consciousness."

- Charles Fillmore, (1854-1948)

Chapter 1

Developing a Mystic Consciousness

"You have not chosen me, but I have chosen you." John 15:16

In this day and age, people are seeking curiosity and a higher spirituality in their life. It appears they are trying to develop a deeper appreciation and awareness of their spiritual self. Most people are searching for a "mystical consciousness." Yet, even though they do not even have this concept in mind, they have a sense of this awareness within a closer walk with Thee. Nevertheless, seekers attend churches, church schools, on-line studies, classes, read books, learn about the wisdom of the ancient sages, and attend universities to seek a deeper understanding. The purpose of this Mystic book is to shed insights and information to help one to "develop a mystic consciousness" and practice it. With that intention in mind, a person will come to understand more fully how to truly walk closer with their Higher Power.

In Charles Fillmore's book, *The Revealing Word* (1959), a mystic is defined as "One who has an intimate first-hand acquaintance with God; a man of prayer." In the same book, (p. 41), consciousness means "the sense of awareness, of knowing." Jesus was the greatest mystic of all ages. Fillmore is the co-founder of the Unity movement.

The founder of Religious Science and author of *The Science of Mind*, Ernest Holmes (1938) defines a mystic as one who uses direct contact with the Divine and should not be confused with a psychic. A mystic has a sense about them that they pick up the presence and thoughts of the Universal God, not another person's thoughts. This truth is the same as mystics throughout the ages of time. It does not change. Psychics tend to not have the same experiences as another and they see through their own perception, influences, psychic senses, nonphysical agencies, and impressions. Each psychic has a different opinion about various events and happenings. A mystic's life may be getting away from the world, a detachment of emotional sense. Marsha Sinetar (1996), a well-known writer on the life of mystics, believed mystics live a contemplative and simple life that corresponds with the term called "purification." Now, you may have a better understanding of the position and posture of a mystic.

While you have the earnest need to draw closer to the Universal Spirit, you may be considering applying the physical and mystical meditation of yoga to improve your overall physical, emotional, spiritual and mental self. With that concept in mind, you may have been told about many myths associated with yoga. Hopefully, after you read this work, it will dispel your fears that may be associated with these falsehoods and help you to understand how yoga contributes to the overall well-being of any person, regardless of their spiritual or moral beliefs.

One of yoga's major falsehoods in Western society is that in order to practice yoga, you must follow a certain eastern religion or faith. The truth is, regardless of a person's spiritual beliefs, anyone can practice yoga. Yoga does require one to worship any particular Deity or a Divine Universal God. Yoga simply teaches beliefs, a system of healthy living. The practice of yoga encourages its participants to practice meditation, silence, tolerance and goodwill toward all things on this planet. Students of yoga are also encouraged to exercise forgiveness and apply love to all mankind, as do traditional and non-traditional religions.

Seeking a Higher Spirituality

In the quest of one's search for what is missing in their lives, an intimate inner knowing is present. Consequently, it is usually a personal relationship with their God. The seeker can gain a self-awareness that has not been developed before. Once a person opens their soul and integrates this knowledge, they can develop a keener spiritual awareness of a Higher Power. This process incorporates an inner knowing that God's Spirit and Divine illumination resides inside them. The devotee of a higher consciousness practices a salute of being unattached to the outer world; stillness, a silence, a spiritual practice; mental prayer and meditation. These are forms of spiritual disciplines taught in martial arts, monasteries, solitude, yoga, convents, Reiki, and various religious schools. For a person to develop and achieve stillness and silence, they must be taught to center themselves, to go within. To accomplish this, one must let go of their conscious thoughts and turn their fears inward to the heart center. As one journeys on their personal spiritual path to a new beginning, the soul will travel in humility, trust, and faith in a Higher Power. Most have an inner question, "What is happening to my soul?" Then, they do not rush the answers. They need to become still to hear or sense the feelings. Many say, "I feel different." This is the perfect time to tune in again and ask, "What are the needs of my soul?" They sense and feel feelings that they had not felt before as they advance higher in levels of spirituality. There is no short cut into a "spiritual awakening." One must go through it. A few will continue to encounter inner pains, distractions, illness, uncomfortable feelings, fears and will desire a blueprint to follow. However, if one would study and then follow the blueprints and guidance left for us by the mystic and other ancient sages and faithful spiritual followers, they would be enlightened by their determination and fortitude. Nevertheless, in the act of entering stillness and silence, the soul goes through withdrawals, experiencing resistance and the shedding of negative ego patterns that have been developed. Layer upon layer, the patterns shed themselves down to the very core of a person. Then, they do not know what they believe or trust. This is the information that is timely insights, presented here for my metaphysics readers to help them understand what they may be feeling. If only one can make it through the "darkened times." There is dark and the light, both to assist one along the spiritual path.

Looking to the Saints

In the contents of this book, there are several mystics who lived between the thirteenth and twentieth centuries. The book of Luke from the Holy Bible says, "For unto whomsoever much is given, of him shall be much required" (Luke 12:48). These people are mystics, who lived a life dedicated to their God. They were dedicated to their spiritual experience. It was taught one-on-one.

This text's focus will be primarily on Saint Teresa of Avila and Saint John of the Cross. These individuals are identified as mystics because they are persons of faith who believed that the awareness of spiritual truth and communion with God could be attained through personal experience, dedication, intuition, or insight. Saint Teresa (1515-1582) was a sixteenth century Roman Catholic nun. She was a mystic, a teacher, and a Spanish author who sought to reform the Church. Her mystical experiences did not happen until she was nearly forty years old. Even though she was a dedicated nun and elected official, she had charm, lots of humor, was a very good cook, and a wonderful conversationalist. She was a wonderful business woman and her focus remained on her inner passions of poverty as a contemplative life, just like her role model, Saint Clare of Assisi (1195-1253). Everyone who seeks a better spiritual way should have a spiritual role model. For example, Saint Clare of Assisi also set and wrote her own rules three years before her death. Around 1247, she endorsed poverty by starting the Poor Ladies' Rule, a charity. She devoted her teachings to assist the poor and needy. One of the strong points in her teachings was letting go of negative feelings and the material things of life. In the words of Saint Clare, she instructed all when they prayed to pray with power, to "look to your letting go." "Let go and Let God" may be what the Saint was implying; turning your concerns over to Spirit. One thing that is so different about the writings of Saint Teresa and Saint Clare is that Saint Clare of Assisi wrote to her students in absolute confidence. She knew in her own words that "this pattern of life can work," a vow of poverty. Saint Teresa often experienced inner doubts, even though she "slipped away in her own private chamber," in her own words. She says in the Introduction section of her book, *The Book of My Life*, "You fall to your knees at the alter you keep there ... You feel it coming on, watch in patient fascination as the familiar, mysterious feeling washes over you. It gathers all fragmented parts and lifts you out of yourself." Nonetheless, Saint Clare was an influence on how Saint Teresa implemented the vows of poverty to the monks and nuns (Flinders, 1993).

Our Teacher's from 600 Years Ago

Even the beautiful Saint Teresa was surrounded by the temptations of men. She never blamed men for wanting her attention. Her exhortation was to never displease God. There were many scandals of her and men (Flinders, pp. 155-190). This woman was a profound spiritual teacher, whose books will instruct, inspire, delight souls' paths, as she teaches about her signature "mental prayers" and illuminates anyone who reads her works, especially you. Dear reader, you will see her as a human, dying to herself in order to serve her Beloved. You will learn so much from her and others within this book. I encourage you to buy her book *Teresa of Avila: The Book of My Life*. (2007)

Saint John of the Cross was also from the sixteenth century. He was a Carmelite friar and priest, Spanish poet and Roman Catholic mystic. He was much younger than Saint Teresa. He was old enough to be her son but he was dedicated to her cause and to her soul. He was born in Fontiveros, Spain (a small village near Avila) in 1542. He was kidnapped, imprisoned, and placed in solitary confinement by his superiors for nine months after refusing to follow the orders of his superiors to relocate, allegedly due to his attempts to reform life within the Carmelite order. While being forced to endure physical, emotional, and mental abuse for those nine months, he wrote about being free and escaping to do the work of the Spirit. Saint John of the Cross could identify with the emotional suffering of Saint Teresa and many others, even people today, like you. His greatest work was done in solitude, in prison, and in the silence. As the Saint sat alone, he welcomed those "dark nights" to sense a presence of his God. He penned *Dark Nights of the Soul* (1959) while in prison. He left a blueprint showing how to bring one's self out of the "dark nights of the soul." His works, *Christian Walk Ascent of Mount Carmel* and the *Dark Nights of the Soul*, as a mystic writer is one the grandest literature book components. It is my position to educate *all* who come across my path to the real life of those who truly were followers of their spiritual quest and Beloved God. Most people who desire a "higher calling" think the road is very easy. They must understand it is worth it but it may not be totally easy. If one applies faith and exercises daily in their spiritual walk, the dark nights will become a lighted path and directions will appear.

Do You Know How to Make it Through the Night?

The profound Rev. Michael Beckwith (2008), shares "how to make it through the night." When the time comes for spiritual seekers who are trying to figure out what is going on and they cannot sleep through the night, guidelines and insights are given. To the persons who want to evolve, these instructions are essential to their spiritual growth. This information is necessary to those who are dedicated to their "spiritual practices" and want to become integrated with the Universal God. Seekers should welcome instead of resist the "dark nights." When one resists anything, an inner fight occurs and the days become long. Yes, they should welcome the opportunity to enter the "mystical darkness," but they must understand that this is a time when the senses will be purified and corrected. The ego is shredded and unrobed, torn into pieces of paper to be thrown away into a sea of nothingness. The soul and spirit are torn into rags for a spiritual perfection to be clothed. The nature of spiritual seekers is that all imperfections and disorders go under a microscope by the Universal Creator and removed from the soul. This is by the seeker's choice to become purified. Saint John tells that a spiritual seeker will not enter the second night and the next, until they pass the first test of removing all imperfections and habits. This is the process of "developing a mystic consciousness" to gain enlightenment within one's soul and spiritual path.

In *Bookmark Prayer* of Teresa of Avila states:

> "Let nothing disturb you, nothing frighten you. All things are passing. Everything is changing. God never changes. Patience endurance will attain to all things. Who God possesses, in nothing is wanting; alone God suffices."

A French Carmelite Teacher from the Late 1800's

Saint Theresa of Lisieux was called the "Little Flower of Jesus" (1873-1897). She was a French Carmelite of the late eighteenth century. At age fifteen, she entered the convent. She never left the four walls of her convent. Her Beloved called her to be a nun at age nine. Even at an early age, her spiritual mission was to stand up for social justice and reforms of a devotional "spiritual practice." She, like others, gained support from the readings of Saint John of the Cross. Saint Theresa followed the teaching of Saint Teresa of Avila. In passion, she cared about her sisters as taught by Saint Teresa. She was a "friend in spirit." She died at age twenty-four.

The Woman who Practices Total Surrender

Mother Teresa, known as Agnes at birth, was born in 1910. At age 18, she stood for the suffering of the poor in the world, to a religious and missionary life. At age twelve, she felt, she says, a "gentle call" to a religious and missionary life. She did nothing about her calling for many years. She prayed and thought about the mission for six years. Do we often put off our divine call from God, not acknowledge the call at all, or do we rush it? She said, "YES!" Her religious name became

Teresa. She later picked up the saintly guide, Saint Theresa of Lisieux – "Little Flower of Jesus."

From the book, *A Simple Path*, Mother Teresa asked her confessor for advice about her "call or vocation." She asked, "How can I know if God is calling me?" The confessor told Mother Teresa, "You will know by your happiness. If you are happy with the idea that God called you to serve Him and your neighbor, this will be proof of your vocation. Profound joy of the heart is like a magnet that indicates the path of life one will follow, although the way is full of difficulties." (Vardey, 1997)

Mother Teresa of Calcutta grew in spiritual knowledge from reading Saint Theresa's (her spiritual role model) instructions on how to take care of the poor. While centered on doubts about the afterlife, she reportedly told her nuns, "If you only knew what darkness I am plunged into." At the time of her death, the sisters wrote her words down every day that she spoke. She spoke the word, "Mother, it is the way of spiritual childhood; it is the way of confidence and total abandon. I want to teach them ... to tell them there is only one thing to do here on earth: to cast at Jesus the flowers of little sacrifices, to take Him by caresses; this is the way I've taken Him, and it's for this that I shall be so well received" (Flinders, 1993). Consequently, readers have thought only the mystic lives in a heightened spiritual state at all times and remains there. As we understand it, they too welcome and enter into dark periods in order to reach a closer connection with their God. This was a deep obligation. How often do you enter those dark places?

The popular saint and mystic of the twentieth century was Mother Teresa of Calcutta. She was the founder of the Missionaries of Charity, and known for her works for the poor and the dying. She kept a smile on her face and a positive attitude throughout her lifetime of spiritual work. She took many vows, but one was to remain poor. Within her kingdom, her soul, she faced many doubtful days from 1948 until she died in 1997. Franciscan Friar, Father Benedict Groeschel, who was a friend to Mother Teresa for a large part of her life, tells us, "The darkness left towards the end of her life" (Mother Teresa of

Calcutta, 1985). She teaches that "souls of prayer are souls of great silence."

Mother Teresa thought it was one's duty to work together in an effort to keep an interior of deep silence and thought for their lives. The end result would be an awareness of the Divine Presence for all people everywhere, in their hearts, as well as for the poor people. One of her favorite scriptures on silence is (Hosea 2:16-18), "Behold, I will allure her and will lead her into the wilderness and I will speak to her heart." For those who seek a "mystic consciousness," they do not have to vow to work with the poor or to be poor, depressed, or be isolated unless they choose to do so. One can be a mystic without this undertaking. They can just serve the human race, their family and friends. They do not have to write, teach or minister, but they do have to live in the light of the Universal God. Most choose to give back in Divine importations of art, music, books, seeing after the sick, homeless, orphans, and lonely, etc. There are many who are obliged or led to do this type of compassionate service, but do not know why. It is my mission to educate them on the Divine importations of a mystic life. Mother Teresa counsels her nuns and brethren again from *A Simple Path*: "Take time to be silent, and to contemplate, especially, she said, when you work in big cities." London and New York were a few of her examples for cities that move too fast and were too noisy. She created a Contemplative Sister's home (whose vocation is to pray most of the day) in New York instead of quiet places like the Himalayas. She said, "I felt silence and contemplation were needed more in large cities of the world." Mother always starts her day with prayer in silence, she says, "It is in the silence of the heart that God speaks, God is the friend of silence-we need to listen to God because it's not what we say, but what He says to us, and through us, that matter ..." (pp. 7-9)

Modern Day Teacher

Sylvia Browne, founder and minister of the Society of Novus Spiritus, teaches in her book, *Mystical Traveler* (2008) how to advance

14

spiritually as a "mystical traveler." A "mystical traveler" is one who has already developed their oneness with their Mother and Father God. Often, the "mystical traveler" is called to go wherever God would like them to go. They work a lot behind the scenes to serve others, as well as on the front lines. Countless people on this earth who are seeking a higher enlightenment feel restless until they answer this calling. A few do not even have a name for it. They just feel what they are seeking. Often, they seem to look to other places, things and people for guidance and directions instead of the Universal God. When working with those who are seeking more spirituality, I will offer this insight within this book. I have also felt the need to go here and move there without knowing why. However, once I applied faith, the journey was unveiled as to why. I was there to do a mission for God. Later, in due season, it was revealed (Batey 2009). How often have you felt like you should move?

According to Jim Pym, author of *Listening to the Light* (1999), the Quaker religion uses silent worship for personal prayers along with meditation. The Quaker religion refers to this as "Listening to the Light." With the blueprint the Saints have left over time, the example of holiness for all is attainable. What has been learned inside the silence is a rich knowledge within our own soul. The inner awareness is heightened and treasured. Our role models could not go another way but to the sacred silence; it was their duty (Davis 1990). Through the teachings of these faithful Saints, there are blueprints and guidance to be followed. As a Doctor of Mystical Research, I share the teachings of these mystics in this book - their strengths, challenges, and how their spirituality was enhanced as they became dedicated and followed their Beloved's spiritual work. There are many more mystics that you may choose to learn about, but these are a few who left their imprints within my soul, and now I pray yours.

From the words of Mother Teresa's book, *Total Surrender* (pp. 103-104, 1985):

> "Each one of us will take it as our serious and sacred duty to collaborate with one another in our common effort to

15

promote and maintain an atmosphere of deep silence and recollection in our own lives, conducive to the constant awareness of the Divine Presence everywhere and in everyone, especially in our own hearts and in the hearts of our sister (brothers I added), with whom we live in the poorest of the poor.

To make possible true interior silence, we shall practice silence of the ears, eyes, heart, tongue, and mind. Our silence is a joyful and God- centered silence; it demands of us constant self-denial and plunges us into the deep silence of God where aloneness with God becomes a reality."

Dear, enter into a Silence, yoga, meditation along with prayer, and create a spiritual practice. As part of my spiritual practice, I do Kabbalah yoga. The Jewish word, Kabbalah means "that which is received." You may be wondering, "What is received?" Enlightenment from the Universal God, messages from the inner most part of my soul, my true purpose and destiny, and mystical teachings, are just a few examples. My mind is sharpened and I learn how to adjust the wandering mind and body to eliminate distractions, which will transform challenges and obstacles. As I stay in this Kabbalah yoga practice, I feel gratitude for all things in my world. Then, I am guided along my spiritual journey. The road is not always clear and bright, however, as I renew my mind, it starts anew. Flexibility is created into my body, mind and spirit.

_____

_____

_____

_____

_____

_____

Chapter 2

Getting to Know You!

"Know Thyself" -Socrates (49-399 BC)

As one searches, looking to receive insights while traveling on their spiritual runway of life, they often seek unknowingly, a Higher Consciousness and heightened awareness. They can achieve this development by putting a spiritual practice in place and exercising a mystical meditation and prayer. From the words of a New Thought mystic, Charles Fillmore:

"Know thyself", "know who and what you are, where you came from, what you are doing here and where you are going. If you want to know all this, meditate on the "I AM" (2005, p.38). The Way-Shower, Jesus taught, when this type of mystical prayer happens within the silence of our mind, heart, and contemplation, one communes with our Higher God Mind. But first, a person must shut the door to the outside world and only then can one enter into true contemplation and silent meditation."

Seek Understanding

Saint Francis, a thirteenth century mystic, taught this prayer: "Seek first to understand, then to be understood." You are asking how? How well do you know yourself, my dears? Do you know who you are in relation to the Universal God? What is your purpose that you were born to do? What gifts and talents did you come in this world to share? Genesis 1:27 states, "In the beginning, "God created man in his own image, in the image of God created he him; male and female created he them." Unity Teacher and Minister, Eric Butterworth, taught in his book, *Spiritual Economics*, that he agrees with that Bible verse. He discusses how we are all children of the Universe. Do you feel or know that statement to be true for you? Each of us is richly blessed with the fullness of the Universal God. *Who are you?* You are not just the offspring, Butterworth shares, of your parents. You are truly a child of God. A creation of the Infinite source of all our being and you are entitled to the same constant support as the lilies of the fields; he encourages us still from His book: "Consider the lilies of the field, how they grow; they toil not, neither do they spin" (Matthew 6:28). While seeking understanding, one must enter into Quiet Prayer. Understanding comes within your soul; another person cannot give it to you. Position and center your inner being by making Quiet Prayer a part of your spiritual practice. Ask for a change from within your heart and soul. Unite your soul with the Christ the Father within you, or your Higher Power. To understand who you are, you must be willing to conquer all fears and face any self-imposed demons you have created. Make a commitment to enter into the Silence, and then ask the Spirit to bring your fears to the Light of Christ to resolve them. Next, in the Silence of your inner tabernacle, see each one of your fears floating away, one by one. You will find that it is true dwelling in the secret place of the Most High. It is a blissful state that does not require language. You are now ready to move to another level of transformation on your spiritual journey and destiny. In the words of the philosopher, Rumi (1207-1273): "A great silence overcomes me, and I wonder why I ever thought to use language."

Who's There to Assist Us?

Do you know who is there to assist you?

The Holy Spirit abides within us. We also have non-physical teachers, angels, and guides who are assigned to help us on our path while we are here on earth. There are also human beings assigned to us, who assist in our learning of life's lessons. They impart wisdom along our journey and provide support when we need it most. An example of this would be the spiritual leaders, metaphysical life coaches, and teachers at your churches, synagogues, spiritual centers, temples, internet, meetings, iPod, or your home. They are there to offer guidance and to help direct your spiritual path. We are each other's "earth angels" on a Divine mission to assist when we hear the call. However, our hearts must be open to receiving the message. To receive is an act of will. Our free will (our birthright) allows us to choose what we do or do not receive. If we seek, we will find. If we knock, the doors of understanding shall be opened. If we ask for knowledge and wisdom in faith, it shall be given. Saint Teresa of Avila has been the most non-physical angel for me. The books written by her over 600 years ago about her strange prayer life and her penmanship helped me to discover the needs of my soul. This enlightening teacher consciously dedicated herself to helping others know their individual souls and God, which she declared as part of her life's purpose. Even so, she thought it was our divine appointment for this life for us to know God. Gary Zukav tells us in his book, *Seat of the Soul*, (pp. 98-99), "Our non-physical teachers bring us closer to the knowledge of our soul; they impart their knowledge by listening and by giving instruction." He tells us that teachers are more involved than guides. They are impersonal energies that we personalize and feel an intimate relationship with. We should intentionally accept their guidance and then give thanks for all the help we receive from both our guides and our teachers. They are constantly available to serve us and will reveal themselves within varying manifestations and spiritual communications. In the *Seat of the Soul*, (pp. 98-100), Zukav tells us:

> "Non-physical Guides help us when we have important tasks such as writing, putting something together creating, or speaking ... The road to your soul is through your heart. When we close the door to our feelings, we close the door to the vital currents that energize our thoughts and actions."

How open is your heart to your feelings? If it is not open, then it is blocking the flow of Spirit and Life. Information is being sent to your heart from Spirit. Do you know who created you and who you are?

Rumi (1207- 1203) also reminds us to: "Be empty of worrying. Think of who created us."

Lay Down Your Masks

Can you take the time to identify any mask you are wearing?

Is your identity enmeshed in the money you make, the car you drive, the clothes you wear, your education, your job, or the place you worship? Do you feel confused or depressed? Do you use food or drugs to self-medicate your inner pain? Where is the big man in the sky? What does the Universal God mean to me? Is God mad at you? Do you blame others for your mishaps, hold onto past hurts, failures, and missing the mark (sin). Whatever mask we wear, we must identify and remove them, and then realize who we are once they are gone, replacing them with something positive.

"The most important kind of freedom is to be what you really are. You trade in your reality for a role. You trade your sense for an act. You give up your ability to feel, and in exchange, put on a mask. There can't be any large-scale revolution until there's a personal revolution, on an individual level. It's got to happen first inside. You can take away a man's political freedom and you won't hurt him, unless you take away his freedom to feel. That can destroy him. That kind of freedom can't be granted. Nobody can win it for you." - Jim Morrison (1943-1971) Member of the American Band, *The Doors.*

Seek to understand what mask you have been wearing. Who are you really? Ask your soul what your needs are and what is it yearning for? "For there is nothing covered, that shall not be revealed; neither hid, that shall not be known" (Luke 12:2).

Remember, "This above all: to thine own self be true. And it must follow, as the night the day. Thou canst not then be false to any man." –William Shakespeare, *Hamlet,* (1564-1616)

Have you asked yourself why you are here? Try, in your silence meditations and spiritual practices, to get that question answered. I would like to recommend the book by Rabbi David C. Cooper, *God is a Verb: Kabbalah and the Practice of Mystical Judaism*, as well as the DVD *Kabbalah Yoga (www.kabbalahyoga.com)*. I know that your real self and purpose will be revealed. In closing, Phyllis Adair Robinson created a poem I would like to share with you:

"Who Am I?

First, I am a child of God
I am spirit and matter formed physically
Into a woman and a man
I am many faces
I can do many things
I have been a child to experience many overwhelming events from the past
I am a Dreamer who faith has raised me from my circumstances and survived
I am a sister, friend, wise gentle soul,
Sensitive and caring
I am an artist who has painted many pictures in my mind
And on the canvas of my life and others
I am now a middle-aged adult soul searching, seeking my special place inexistence on this place called Earth."
-Phyllis Adair Robinson (1960-present)

Namaste'

_____

_____

_____

Chapter 3

Spiritual Literature

"The spiritual life does not remove us from the world but leads us deeper into it." - Henri J. M. Nouwen (1932-1996)

Seekers of enlightenment are looking for a higher spiritual awakening into a higher calling of devotion to their Creator; they are looking for blueprints. Just like a builder who builds homes or buildings, they too follow a blueprint. As a result, as the builder follows clear directions, the project is completed. However, most people only know God the Creator through another person or media – parents, close relatives, minister, or a book. Mystics are those who are called to experience God in sense, feeling, and the wisdom of Spirit first-hand, not far away in a distance. Authors Ronald Hennies and Sonia Weiss (2004) describe it this way: "*a mystic is one who practices or believes in mysticism.*" Mathew 22:14 states, "*For many are called, but few are chosen.*" Everyone on earth is called to understand and integrate with Spirit; it is a personal choice. Spirit teaches mystics on a deep level within their consciousness. Mysticism is found in every religion, culture and age on this earth from the North, South, East and West of the continent. Thus, faithful "mystical travelers" are led to move and go here or there without knowing why. Nonetheless, they later learn why they were called to serve mankind and develop an inner knowing. These people are not afraid to dare to uncover their different spiritual paths.

Mother Teresa was a high school teacher before answering her call to God. The call came on the 10th of September 1946, the day their Catholic church celebrates "*Inspiration Day.*" From the book, *The Joy of Loving*, she is on a train to another city when she is told by Jesus: "*I want you to serve Me among the poorest of poor"* (Chalika and Le Joly, 2000). The authors claim this movement and encounter with Jesus changed her life.

Sylvia Browne describes in her book, *Phenomenon* (2005), the "mystical traveler said to God about their soul's journey is, 'Whatever in this Universe you needs me, I'll willing go.' Mystical Travelers ... devote themselves to maintaining the divine spiritual connection between us and God as a thriving, viable force." Browne continues, "Mystical Travelers have a peaceful acceptance of sacrifice and discomfort when it comes to going forth with their mission on earth" (p. 190). This person is often likened unto Martin Luther, the father of the Protestant Reformation in Germany, Mother Teresa of Calcutta, and Thomas á Kempis, an Augustinian monk to name a few (Foster and Smith, 1990). This may be your path. This poignant information will be valuable to them, knowing that their attachment is to God, not to persons, places, and things.

Listening to the Universal God

Various times, people are often pursued by others to seek other destinies, not to fulfill their spiritual paths - their inner calling from the Universal God. Nonetheless, there have been those who neglect to listen to a prompting of their soul's nudging from Spirit. Hence, procrastination happens by making their passions, desires, and goals a priority in their lives. Thus, they are afraid of making a commitment to prioritize spiritual goals, allowing fears to prevent them from saying "Yes" to the Universal God. Once an individual can identify their fears, overcome them, and subsequently decide what they are willing to leave behind, then growth can occur in their life. Numerous seekers are so afraid of losing out on material things and going places, that they forgo the spiritual journey. Therefore, to make it easy, there are blueprints available from the Saints who have gone before us in this life.

When seekers are unsettled in their spiritual life, their spirit and souls are drawn to another level, growth, or stage of spiritual devotion. This process may leave them feeling uncomfortable and unsettled. When that feeling happens, the masterpiece of mystical literature and blueprints of the sixteenth century, Carmelite Mystic Priest, Author Saint John of the Cross and others may come as a guide. In his book, *Dark Nights of the Soul*, Saint John equates two different phases - the first phase is a purification process; the second is spiritual. This means as one develops and enhances their devotion of spirituality, they begin to become purified, cleansed, and then their spiritual eyes are awakened. In one stanza of *Dark Nights of the Soul*, he writes: "On a dark night, kindled in love with yearnings - oh happy chance! - I went forth without being observed, my house being now at rest." (p. 33) The house was his soul!

You Can Achieve Spiritual Liberation

Accordingly, the author of *Spiritual Liberation*, Michael Beckwith shares insights from a chapter in his book, (p. 237): "As one can see, he (St. John) delighted on the chance to go into a 'dark night of the soul'." However, this period may last for years, one night, or weeks, and one may feel that there is no ending. Seekers seek answers to their new challenge, but no one can clearly give them an answer. After continuing their "spiritual practices," they sense that they are still disconnected to their Universal God, but they are not. While in that activity, we become teachable, reachable, cleansed from our own thoughts, and humbled that we do not know everything about the spiritual journey. Beckwith calls this "positive ignorance." A removal of false ego is taking place and lifted from our levels of consciousness. This is a part of the spiritual awareness journey. Despite the fact that one is feeling unsure of their connection to their Beloved God, the inner question should be asked (which we learn from Beckwith), "How may I be of service to God?" (pp. 239-240)

The remarkable Spanish Mystic nun, author and teacher, Saint Teresa of Avila, was known by her Bishops for her unusual "prayer life," left books for seekers. Her "spiritual practices" were so unheard of that her Bishops commanded her to write books as instructions on prayer. She did not want to write. She said: "Let the learned men who have studied do the writing. I am a stupid creature and don't know what I am saying ..." Once they knew her prayer life was real, she was put under many tests to prove herself and that her actions were not from the devil. Saint Teresa was obedient to the call from her Bishops, no matter what she felt about her own limitations to write about her spiritual life as a guide book. One of the main themes in her books is how she faced doubts, fears, self-esteem issues, isolation and depression. This happened, even though she was in prayer and meditation most of her day. Her Bishops did not understand the wanderings of her soul and neither did she. She went to seek help to understand but they did not have the insight to help her. No one else would try to help her until Saint John of the Cross escaped from prison after nine months and ran into her. She wished that someone could explain why she was feeling the way she did. Here was a devotee of God, who still experienced human struggles and inner limitations like people today and even faced moments of insanity. Yet, no one was able to give her insights into the nature of her problems until she met Saint John of the Cross. He told her she had entered the "*Dark Nights of the Soul.*" Then, he became her confessor and devoted friend. Within her many books, she tells the nuns and the monks, "Their only destiny in this life is to know God and to know their soul." It is my goal as a writer, teacher and Doctor of Metaphysics to help you understand that this true concept - that once you know God and understand the yearnings of your soul, then you can step into a deeper spiritual practice without fear.

Transforming Divine Importations

During Saint Teresa's dedication to her "spiritual practices," she was able to transform her mysticism into the Divine importations of art, poetry, music, prayer, meditation, and dance. In one of her well-known mystical literary works, *Interior Castle* (1946), she had a vision and saw a diamond with many shapes and facets. It was a castle with many chambers and rooms, which she likened to the soul. Then, she likened her thoughts about the scripture, "In My Father's house are many mansions; if it were not so, I would have told you. I go to prepare a place for you." (John 4:2) That vision showed her the center is the chief area where the Spirit lives in the castle and the most secret things pass between God and the soul. Dear reader, I would like you to understand how the answers are within their soul in the center of their being, not outside. There are seven rooms she sees in the castle, which she names in order to reach the center. Each room unfolds the stages of a spiritual awakening for reaching the center, where the Beloved lived, and then enlightenment is reached. Each room has a meaning for progression or "soul clarity," then a completion for the integration of the Divine Union (Myss, 2001).

Sacred Contacts, an insightful book written by Carolyn Myss (pp. 79-80), set forth another literary mystic's work by Evelyn Underhill, as she writes about the "dark nights of the soul" in her book, *Mysticism* (1993). Underhill has condensed the "enlightenment process" into five stages: Awakening, Purification, Illumination, The Dark Nights of the Soul, and Divine Union. A Divine Union is the last room where higher spiritual devotion integration is started between the soul and the Beloved. At this stage, the light of God resides within them. The goals are to light up a person's entire soul and consciousness. The Divine Union is felt after a period of the "dark nights of the soul" is gone. You cannot run away from this act if one is seeking a higher spirituality; it is an ongoing process until completed.

Thomas Moore, author of *Care of the Soul* (1994), has insightful blueprints on the care of one's soul today while entering the "dark nights of the soul." There can be a "Gift of Depression" that can enhance a person's soul and life. Depression is a psychological sickness;

a dark night is a spiritual experience or trial; these are Moore's findings. Thus, a spiritual response is needed for "dark nights," not a therapeutic one. One may try to get this lesson over with quickly or do away with the darkness, but lessons may not be learned. Changes within one's consciousness and soul may be overlooked. The "dark nights" are transformative times for reshaping one's spiritual path and soul. Many have felt uncomfortable as mentioned. This is a transformational period. They may feel isolated. This is when metaphysical coaching or consulting can assist, which is what I want to share with my readers. Even after they have seen a medical doctor, many seem to still be in a state of depression with no spiritual answers, even though they have been faithful to their spiritual growth and beliefs. During this type of soul transformation, many may feel isolated, dull or numb. They enter therapy or seek other professional help from a Minister, only to find they have no answers, which is the same practice Saint Teresa of Avila did for many years. There are scores of human beings who live in monasteries with walls and without walls. These are not just monks or nuns, but everyday people who experience inner struggles daily. The conflict of doubt is present as well, even with their dedication to the Universal God. As one develops and understands a "mystic consciousness," they are able to adjust their daily routine automatically for a positive result (Davis, 1990).

When creative individuals are writing, painting, songwriting, contemplating a speech, or conducting research in order to share information with others, they are often led by Spirit to enter into a period of isolation and silence. This is normally done away from people, places and things that would distract them from producing an inspiring effect. This is usually when creativity emerges. Several experience these events as gifts from God, shining through the darkness into their inner light within their souls. This period should be welcomed no matter how uncomfortable, for the discomfort is only temporary. This is an important concept that I want to bring into reality for my readers of metaphysics. Most are afraid to stay in that place. Staying connected to a Higher Power or God-self, no matter how one is feeling is the key. Replacing any negative thoughts that will creep into the subconscious with gratitude will help. By reading the literature of the mystics and sages that have gone before, practicing a spiritual practice and centering your thoughts in a positive manner, will result in shedding the ego.

Holistic Bodywork

Within this metaphysical writing, I would like you, the reader, to understand the benefits of holistic bodywork as you integrate the masterpiece of mystical knowledge of the saints. There are five major branches of yoga, along with a mystic meditation coupled with massage for releasing body tension. *Hatha* is the path of energy, with emphasis on energetic balancing. *Bhakti* is the path of devotion, emphasizing worship. *Karma* is the path of action, with emphasis on service. *Jnana* is the path of wisdom, focusing on self-inquiry. *Raja* is the royal path, with emphasis on meditation. I will share more on the five major types of yoga later in this book. The majority of people that I life-coach and or/provide massage therapy to, who are trying to re-create their lives, could benefit from this practice. After dealing with a full range of life's ups and downs, such as a nine-to-five structured corporate employment, mid-life crises', job losses, health issues, loss of income, life after divorce or death of a loved one, they are anxious to step into their desired destiny such as writing a book, creating songs, or beginning a new project. These people face fear, doubt and worry. Thus, by integrating the modality of yoga and the mental discipline of meditation into their lives, they will be able to release their tensions and learn "how to" relax their minds and allow the Universal Mind of God to direct their paths. As a life-coach, I have been working with individuals who have not been able to achieve their full potential because they were not implementing a "spiritual practice" of yoga and other things. Many people fear the unknown and yoga will help them unleash their inner vision with ease and grace. I feared the unknown so much after my twenty-one year marriage ended.

I too resisted moving forward. Have you? People also tend to wear masks in their daily lives. We ultimately learn to be dishonest, even with ourselves, in our innermost secret dialogue. I admit I was fearful and doubted myself. I put on many masks of being calm and all together. However, by refusing to acknowledge the truth and putting on these masks, we often complicate the situation and increase our stress within our body and soul. I stopped attending a place of worship. I stepped back from truth, yoga, and a communion with Spirit. However, the Spirit never left me, even though I ate all the wrong things for my body, mind and spirit and gained weight. We set self-imposed limitations on ourselves out of fears that stem from negative emotions that exist within our lives. We must battle against these limitations every day. In order to battle against these emotions, we must arm ourselves with the necessary inner tools, of a spiritual practice and the knowledge that no limitations exist when you walk with the Universal Mind of God. Winning such battles is the only way to reach our divine destinies and becoming center in thoughts while reading the literature of mystics or the sages.

In *Letters of Myrtle Fillmore* (1936), co-founder of the Unity Movement, Fillmore writes these insightful words to followers around the globe:

> "We are taught to center our thoughts within, and then to shut the door; that is, to close our mind to all other thinking and think about God and His goodness and wonderful love; to pray to God in secret, in 'the secret place of the Most High and all things needful will be added."

Chapter 4

Monastery Without Walls

"Silence is the language of God" - Swami Sivanada (1887-1963)

Dr. Bruce Davis, therapist and author of *Monastery Without Walls* (1990) writes: "Silence and prayer are like two best friends who take each other on all kinds of journeys. Through prayer we find the hidden rooms and gardens of silence within us." Saint Teresa speaks about the seven rooms, the chambers or dwelling places within one's soul, and likens it to the mansions Jesus spoke about. In John 2:6, the Holy Bible, tells of the dwelling places, an exterior wall of the temple where there were many chambers the ministers used for counseling others. Could it be that we are to enter into our chamber in a silence and minister to our inner being? Ernest Holmes (1998) states that the word *silence* is one of the most misunderstood words used by metaphysicians. People often believe they must go to a place and do something to achieve silence. There are no special rules to enter into silence; it starts within one's soul as a desire. As one enters the "inner tabernacle or chamber" of their soul, the process begins as they shut the door to their mind and soul. This is not the only way seekers can enter the silence - they may use prayer and meditation, singing, yoga or a form of physical exercising, journaling, dancing or reading uplifting books, etc. Communion with Spirit begins a unity of awareness within one's soul. For those seeking a higher spiritual awareness, there is nowhere to go. Society has taught we must go here and there. It is simply within one's soul. The Gospel of Matthew 6:6 is one of my favorite verses in the Holy Bible: "But you, when you pray, go into your room, and when you have shut the door, pray to your Father who is in the secret place; and your Father who sees in secret will reward you openly." One may think of the secret place as an inner chamber. Psalms 91:1, David tells us, "He who dwells in the secret place of the Most High shall abide under the shadow of the Almighty." Charles

Fillmore has said it so well in the *Revealing Word* (p. 154),"To enter it is to turn the attention from the without to the within," tapping into the inner consciousness of man or woman. Then, really shut the door into the minds, thoughts, and every distracting inner disturbance.

Why not try *Raja* yoga, the king of all yoga poses, with an emphasis on meditation. This form of yoga is activated by turning inward for a higher degree of understanding and meditation. It is the royal union to the mind that enters into meditation to create deeper development with a Higher Consciousness. The psycho-physical structure is one of the challenging structures for people of the West who seek yoga practices because this practice calls for deeper self-discipline, care of the body, health related issues, restraints on intoxicants, speech and mind. Westerners face many addictions and obsessions; this practice leads to a tranquil inner and outer life. Does your life need a balance or grounding? (Feuerstein and Bodian 1993)

Interior Silence

Contemplative prayer is a practice that creates an interior silence within oneself. It is a form of meditation that creates an interior silence. Saint Teresa of Avila taught contemplative or mental prayer to her nuns and monks. While in stillness and a quiet posture of mental prayer, integration starts within the body, mind and soul where God's spirit resides. The stillness and quiet prayer is translated as entering into contemplative prayer - "Pray without ceasing" (1 Thessalonians 5:17-18). Jim Pym (1999) admonishes, "We sometimes look elsewhere for guidance." Many people, who are seeking a "mystic consciousness," think that contemplative prayers are too simple as a way of listening to Spirit. As spiritual beings living on this earth, we talk too much and listen too little to Spirit's promptings. There are many interruptions and distractions. Therefore, one fails to be centered, relaxed and open to hear their Beloved's call. Individuals seeking to develop a "mystic consciousness" must learn to surrender. Pym advises "to go to worship and honestly enter into a contemplative prayer to Creative

35

Intelligence." He also shares, once contemplative prayer is done, God's presence will affect the Spiritual life of the seeker more than any other "spiritual practice." Even so, there are a few who remain in doubt, fear, distraction, and inner pain who desire a spiritual blueprint to follow. Yet, there are many mysticism literary works to follow and guide those who seek spiritual heights. As noted in this book, the mysticism experience knows no boundaries, languages or culture - it can be for you!

Johnnie Colemon (2009) wrote: "Through prayer and meditation and the Silence, we connect with God, the Source of all power, and give thanks for the awareness of our oneness with Him. Prayer is the avenue through which we attain power." The seeker desires a higher union with the Source of all power and will then gain inner power and connection.

The Voice of the Teacher – The First Door

A known fact about the teacher from nearly 600 years ago, Saint Teresa, a devotee of God, was that her limited abilities were self-claimed. Yet, in 1970, Pope Paul VI gave her the title of "Doctor of the Church." This compassionate, humble spirited woman and her dedication enabled her to accomplish higher levels of spiritual work and growth. She left many blueprints for mystical seekers.

Nevertheless, we are focusing here on her blueprints of *Interior Castle*. In one of her many visions, she describes the scene of seeing a diamond with many shapes and facets. It was a castle with many rooms, which she likens to the human soul. Within the center of the soul was the Chief area where the Beloved God lived. The most secret things pass between God and the soul. Prayer and Meditation is the first room. Prayer and meditation opens the door to wonderful gifts from the Universal God. The first key or door must remain closed, and then Spirit can enter and stay. She believed that souls are so busy in the outside world that God cannot get in. This was her theory over 600 years ago and is still true today. As prayer and meditation are developed, this could become a contemplative mental prayer inside the soul and not spoken out loud. This key or door is where communion with the Beloved starts a sharing between friends. Saint Teresa, after her first rapture, heard the words of her Beloved, "No longer do I want you to converse with men, but with angels" (Avila and Peers 1946). As she wrote, the Bishops knew that she was under fire because of raptures and visions, yet she wrote for the antagonistic audience, most commonly, the Dominicans. They were suspicious of mental prayer, thinking it was a way of avoiding the hierarchy of the Church. Yet, she had determination. I would like to ask you, how many times have you not been understood because of your prayer life and closeness to your Beloved? Prayer starts the mystical life. "Contemplation may also be defined as a loving wisdom which tastes God perfect." - Francois Malaval (1627-1719)

 Bhakti yoga is a branch of yoga that assists in activating a path of devotion and a focus on worship. This is a process that is done from the mind to the heart, with an emphasis on love. Love is the highest vibration on earth. Do you desire a transcending deeper walk with your Deity? There are no congregations, ministers, or religious creed to follow or pledge to with this type of yoga. You integrate this practice with love, prayer and meditation (Feuerstein and Bodian 1993).

Room Two

 A Spiritual Practice can advance a "mystic consciousness" as one attunes to their Higher Power daily. Saint Teresa's "spiritual practice" consisted of contemplation, prayer and meditation, listening to sermons, writing, dancing, edifying conversations, good company, and reading uplifting books. She created blueprints and tools to teach her students about prayer, resisting temptation, and staying connected with the Divine. Once the spiritual seeker seeks a deeper "mystic consciousness," they are often confronted with opposition, distraction, or difficulties. Saint Teresa informs her students to resist the increased temptations, recognizing that we have the spiritual tools to combat them. A "spiritual practice" is personal insurance for their life. This second key or door must be completed before one can enter another room and stay. Do you have a "spiritual practice" that you have in place? "We are not forced to take wings to find Him, but have only to seek solitude and to look within ourselves." (Saint Teresa 1515-82)

For the person who is busy, physically active and desires to unite with the Universal God, *Hatha* yoga is for you. Do you need energetic balancing? In the Hindu text, there is a Chakra system called the seven psychic system locations within the body. They are located from the spine to the crown of the head. When *Hatha* yoga is practiced along with meditation, the Chakra's ancient systems of India are receptive and energies are released within the body (Anodea and Vega p. 262). *Hatha* yoga is forceful. It creates an arousal within the body.

Room Three

The Exemplary Life, the key or door to perfect a prayer life, a higher standard of virtue. Accordingly, Saint Teresa taught that the soul has not yet experienced the full love of Spirit when first entering this room. Saint Teresa warns, as does the Bible, "Trust in the Lord with all thine heart; and lean not unto thine own understanding" (Proverbs 3:5). One should remember that even though they open the door with the key, they must put action behind the act, along with trusting a power that is higher than them. Then, once they experience the fulfillment of the stage or level, they are permitted to move on to another room. The first three rooms were dwelling places within the soul for the start of a beginning or a phase to develop a mental prayer.

Room Four

A Promise to Marry - the key or door is where the mystic life begins. In truth, the Universal Creator is one's first Spiritual Soul Mate. Prayer (desire) of a union (marriage) with God is the key used for entry into living the mystic life. This is a time for a courtship or

long-term dating. A transition or change from one phase into a supernatural place is a prayer of quiet, "Wherein lies the greatness of thy love, O lover?" My love is great in that I have no art therein."
 - Ramon Lull (c. 1232-1315)

Room Five

The Spiritual Betrothal procession by God. This is where one learns to surrender to the personal will of God. Ultimately, your personal self-will merges into the Universal Creator's Will. This is an important key or door for entry. Our desires become the Beloved's Will only in the fifth room. One must die to self will and infuse their thoughts with contemplation, a prayer of union to Christ, a death of the old soul.

Room Six

The Purification stage is where the Lover and the Beloved grow in love in this room. This stage of a mystic is the purification and illumination. Most do not want to go into this room because it does not feel comfortable. It is too dark. One feels the insecurities and experiences the "dark nights of the soul" that Saint John wrote about. One of the greatest fears is that the person is alone and that the Creator is not with them. This is not true. It is a time for deepening one's spiritual awareness and letting go of the false ego. Then, the illumination (the light of God) occurs while this process is going on - then the "dark nights of the soul." A rebirth occurs; a newness after the spiritual torment and a preparation of the last stage.
Jnana yoga is the path of wisdom, focusing on the self. This practice opens the intellectual mind as well as a path of discernment and wisdom for those seeking questions about life. The ultimate purpose is for a sage to reach a higher consciousness with God, and for intuition to come easily into the mind faculty; nonetheless, one will gain a mystical experience (Feuerstein and Bodian 1993). The mind of the

yogi is the true discipline in this branch, focusing on detachment, self-discipline, longing for freedom, breathing exercises, contentment, hearing the truth, reflection upon the truth, and meditation. This truth is discovered by knowledge and practice, not rituals and ceremonies. One of the benefits of *Jnana* yoga is the right-thinking for daily living. Along with that concept, openness and removing blocks that have clouded a person's consciousness are also emphasized. This allows the mystical mysteries that have been hidden within the mind to come to the forefront and flow, which in turn, allows the truth to be discovered, thereby bolstering the chance for better living.

Room Seven

After the "dark nights of the soul," the last key or door is the Divine Union or a dwelling place - The Spiritual Marriage. A complete transformation has been achieved and there is perfect peace. This is the highest stage of the Divine Call or Union where you integrate and dwell with the Beloved. Saint Teresa of Avila taught that wisdom is achieved through humility, detachment, and suffering. She wanted the nuns and monks to understand the wisdom of the soul as they move through each room to finally arrive at the center of one's being. Whenever one gets distracted, or lost, just return back to the first room and start all over. This is good advice from someone who has been there and lived a "mystic consciousness." Teresa is writing about her own experiences. She shows up as a spiritual writer, now in full possession of her knowledge around age sixty-two. Before that, her "spiritual practice" was deeply under fire by her Bishops. A couple years before her death, she is more at peace and confident in her calling to write and do her spiritual work to reform orders. I highly recommend her last book, *Interior Castle*. This is the information that seekers are looking for when they are called to walk a higher, devoted, spiritual life. Most seekers are going through a spiritual and personal transformation. However, they do not understand their feelings of what is occurring. As a Doctor of Metaphysics, I love sharing these insights into this "mystic consciousness" by developing this book for you! "He that seeks no witness for himself without has clearly committed himself wholly unto God." - Thomas A. Kempis (c.1379-1471)

Mystic Archetypes Identified

The word "archetypes" is Greek, meaning model, original pattern and characteristic. There are four principal energy companion Archetypes identified, developed, and defined by author and medical intuitive Carolyn Myss, (Myss 2001), whose purpose is to help people understand their sacred purpose in life. The four Archetypes are Child, Victim, Prostitute, and Saboteur. Often, when one does not know their destiny in this life that they have chosen, it leads to disease and other physical illness. But Myss's book, *Sacred Contract* helps enlighten and outlines guides for the twelve different types of Archetype personalities, from myths and cultural teachings throughout the ages of time. We are going to focus on the Mystic Archetype (Myss pp. 397-398), who, while on earth, used their spiritual personal power to help guide others on this earth (pp. 142-163). More people want to become mystical archetypes until they find out the sacrifices, deep dedication and commitments that are required. Then, they want to pass it along to another. Often, people say they have a "mystic" consciousness, ability and talent, yet, they do not know the undergoing of this Call. The spiritual traits of mystics are enticing on the outside. The truth is that one enters most of their day in prayer and meditation, trances, and some unheard practices. They are called to suffer real pain; they are hard workers, and welcome afflictions just like Jesus on the cross. Mystic's die to themselves daily for their Beloved. Myss shares that most people think they are mystics when they meditate once a day, seek a weekend retreat, and/or attend a yoga workshop. This is not the role of a mystic. A mystic is a person who is seeking a higher spiritual awareness, regardless if they live in the West or East, and practice Christian, Judaism, Muslim, Hindu, Zen, Taoism, Sufi, and etc. A

41

mystic does not desire material gain to be noticed by others or personal things. The Archetype pattern of a mystic is one whose manner is one of renunciation and focus-minded, and who does not seek selfish desires of things and ambitions. They are an *Anchorite* model of a mystic type, a person who withdraws from the world to follow a simple path.

An additional characteristic type is a *Hermit*, who seeks a solitary spiritual path, yet this is not always for seeking spiritual awareness or communion. As you can see, the identifying pattern of a mystic is a person who loves being alone. The main objective for the mystic is for their own spiritual progression and knowing their inner awareness has achieved a "higher state of grace of consciousness." Over and over again, mystics may be repeatedly taken advantage of by people who like them physically, mentally, economically, emotionally and sexually. One of the qualities of a mystic who has reached the spiritual enlightenment stage is that they seek to serve others regardless of what they are enduring. The price they pay while serving is shown in blood, sweat and tears (Myss p. 398).

Are You a Mystical Traveler?

Who are mystical travelers? Sylvia Browne (xxii 2008) states they may travel down two paths: a pilgrim or the pioneer. The quiet workers who work behind the scenes to assist others are pilgrims. They adopt pets, older adults and children that are neglected. The pioneers are those like Martin Luther King, who are in the public sight and gain fame for their work. Saint John of the Cross is an example who started spiritual movements of teachers and writers that are called to tell the world a spiritual message. Mission-life entities assist mystical travelers in performing their duties. All are treated equally in the sight of the Universal God. A person is a free agency to spiritually advance more than another; it is left up to the person. People who are mystical travelers are first a mission-life entity. Billy Graham and George Washington were accomplished, mission-life entities. Browne believes that the blacks who were enslaved, as well as the Jews who were put into camps, were first mission- life entities, and later became mystical travelers (xxiv-xxv).

What makes a mystical traveler? In *Mystical Traveler* (pp. 1-45), Browne defines a mystical traveler as "the highest spiritual advancement." You would never know a "mystical traveler" by looking on their outer being. One may be a teacher, nun, monk, minister, rabbi or a quiet saint; that does not guarantee one will be a "mystical traveler." A lot of people wonder if they have to do self-sacrifice, forms of punishments, denials or practice Christian dogma to advance. Within her book, Browne notes countless regular people just simply take an oath to Mother and Father God or the God of the Universe, and then accept the mantle to join forces with the Creator of the Universe to work. This path is not easy, but one will be infused with healing abilities, grace, spiritual knowledge, and be able to speak and write about the journey to assist others on their path. Your knowledge may not be all correct, nonetheless, it will be closer to right than another. There are six levels to develop if one desires to become a "mystic traveler," as defined by Browne (pp. 6, 7, and 9):

1. Feeling the inner call to a higher awareness and height of spirituality. The person may not be aware of what the call is. It starts in the subconscious, sensing that a call is there.
2. Knowing within one's soul that they want to be a "mystical traveler," even though they are not sure what that demands.
3. Not feeling really comfortable about the call as a "mystical traveler" - a wrestling within the soul. One may wonder what this advanced spirituality represents. This assurance may come by infused knowledge.
4. After surrendering to the will of God, the "mystical traveler" receives the mantle. Once this action is taken, there is no turning back. Browne states, "As it is written, so it will be." There is no outside validation at this level – just acceptance of what gifts one has to offer and the meaning behind them.

5. The activation of the gift of the choice to be a "mystical traveler." Wherever God directs you to travel, you will go. Browne believes that this opportunity was agreed upon long before the person, who wears this mantel, came to earth as a "mystical traveler or a mission-life entity."
6. The last state - the graduation - going home to the network and placement. Once orientation is over on the Other Side, then one will go again wherever God desires.

Everyone who comes to earth does not have to become a "mystical traveler." They can have a normal life. Just like there are levels of schooling such as Stanford or a local state college. Once the 'mystical travelers" complete their levels, they will have a gold star where their third eye is. No one will be able to see this marking. The physical make-up is in various form, shape, race, religions, sex, age, creed and sexual preference. They have been throughout this wide universe and continents. Sylvia Browne did not accept her mantle until she was 50 years old, so did I ... It's all in my book, *Poise for the Runway*. (2009)

There are many precious souls spreading the Light of the Universal God in their lifetimes. They are often called "light-workers." However, many still have not attained the knowledge of a "mystic consciousness nor a mystical traveler." Still, many face and experience illness and depression, but they are not down for long. As they progress in life, they receive many blessings, protection, insights, and the gift of prophecy and healing for taking on this mantle and being willing to assist their God. As my gift to this society, I would like to share this information though is not new in the form of a book, so that others can realize who they are as a "mystical traveler and using a mystic consciousness." (pp. 10-11)

Chapter 5

Spiritual Offering

"The worth of love does not consist in high feelings; but in detachment: in patience under trials for the sake of God whom we love. –Saint John of the Cross (1542-1591)

In society today, people are too busy with their daily life. People do not take the time for silence, mystical meditation, mental prayer, yoga, journaling, solitude or contemplated thinking. Most of these things were taught by Saint Teresa. Nor do they seem to be taking time to develop their spiritual perfection. Therefore, they do not even want to learn a better way of living because they think it may take too much time. There are those who are not seeking a higher spiritual awareness in their lives. The gift of silence and self–mastery is lost because people do not take the time for "spiritual practice." Nonetheless, they sense something is missing in their lives. They experience depression, sadness, loss of hope, and do not understand their purpose of life, and then wonder what the "missing link" is. People of today are so preoccupied with the day-to-day work, and gaining material good, that they have forgotten their purpose here on earth. Maybe, they do not even remember it or know it. This would be a good time look for a DVD of Kabbalah yoga, and ask, "What are the needs of your soul?" Then, they often ask, "What am I doing here on earth?" Remember that Kabbalah means, "That which is received." Ask your soul, "What am I to receive?" Reflect on "Who are you?" "Where was my origin?" "Where may I go and how am I to get where I am supposed to go?" In meditation, I can say from experience that Kabbalah yoga is a life-changing adventure.

It has been said that we are infinite, spiritual beings living a human experience. We are body, mind, spirit and soul connected to a Universal God living within us. Here is a question I would like to ask you, "Do you believe the Universal God dwells within you?" If your answer is yes, it is my job to help you understand how to connect spirituality to the presence within your soul. Next, my mission is to help you to understand "how to" develop a "mystic consciousness" and a "spiritual practice" by sharing blueprints left by the mystics before us. For those who say they do not understand how the Universal God could be living within their soul, it is my attempt in this book to help you understand and become educated with this material and other spiritual, literary mystical works.

Do We Have to Understand?

When Saint Teresa started to teach the monks and nuns about how to enter their "interior silence," there were those who had questions, I am sure. "Why do we have to understand this?" they asked. As a recap, even though her Bishops asked her to write about her prayer life, they too had many questions until she passed their inquiry of test. Then, they realized that her spirituality was from her Beloved. Her spirituality was different from theirs and anyone else they knew. One who is seeking a "mystic consciousness" must understand it will not be an easy path, but it will be worth it, as they are married to their Beloved. Therefore, a person who seeks a higher level of spiritual consciousness may enter into the act of silence. Speaking from my own mystical experience and from the readings of the ancient sages and mystics, the soul goes through withdrawals. One may experience resistance and the shedding of negative patterns built into the ego, which developed over the years and perhaps another lifetime. Layer upon layer, the patterns shed themselves down to the very core of one's soul. When the brain becomes still and quiet during silent meditation, the spirit is being renewed, even though it appears nothing is happening. During this process, one may sense a feeling of down and out, loneliness, and grief, like a death is occurring, as if they are being stripped to the very core of their being. At this wilderness time, a shift within ones' consciousness and soul may begin; a new movement - one may not be able to sleep at times. Most people are too afraid to be alone in our rooms within our souls, when the deeper levels of the false ego are holding to ones' perception. Nonetheless, one senses a disrobing that penetrates into their soul and it does not feel good. As one faces something new, one may create a personal ritual and "spiritual practice" to help release negative behavior patterns. This may be the disrobing of false patterns. For example, if one has a false belief system of who they are or what they do for work. Addictive traits indicate a constant need for other people's approval, a belief in or lack of limitations. Then, they have to let go of their large ego, fear, inner loneliness and anything else that no longer serves them. They may have to ask forgiveness from another, who they may have harmed, and gain an understanding of what happened between them. This is in order to clear the mental atmosphere of all persons involved. At home or another location, you can practice a form of yoga, prayer and meditation, journal writing of your feelings, and deep breathing exercises as your "spiritual practice." This will help the mind, body, spirit and soul to become rested and restored. Also, this practice will help remove and release toxic energies from the soul and body. (Batey 2009)

Too Busy?

A mystical truth seeker, Charles Haanel (Hill 2007) taught, "As long as one is busy the Universe cannot express through a person." People are too busy with their plans and purposes. Once one quiets down the senses, seeks inspiration, gains a mental focus within one's soul, and then lives and dwells in the Omnipotence with a clear consciousness, they will find unity. Another mystical truth seeker, Ralph Waldo Trine, in 1897 shares: "If one would enter in quiet silence a few moments of the day, one may not be bothered by distractions and disturbances that will enter into the physical senses." This silence is one's time to be alone with God. An individual may seek a receptive attitude as they calmly, quietly, and expectantly desire for this spiritual realization to break into their soul and take possession of it. We are too busy in this life with the negative chatter within our souls talking to others. A few are addicted to talking too much for the sake of attention or are over-thinkers. Living in this culture, we can gain control of talking too much, going here and doing this or that. One of the answers is just what the mystic taught, "Being still and knowing that Universal God is in control of this Universe."

Tune into the Infinite Source

As one tunes into the Infinite Source and trusts the wisdom that is given, they can develop a "mystic consciousness" and serve mankind. One should ask for forgiveness of their soul and others, and from others whom they may harbor grudges. This creates an open channel for the soul to receive Divine promptings and guidance. Do you desire to be a channel of good for the Infinite Source? Through the seekers' daily spiritual practice, they will know the needs of their soul. Contemplative thought, fasting, exercising, yoga, reading uplifting books, wholesome foods, journaling, meditation, forgiving others, and mental prayer are the tools that help to deepen spiritual insights and consciousness . This could be what Saint Teresa calls a "spiritual offering."

One cannot go back to the old way of thinking negative thought patterns when seeking to reach a higher spiritual walk and wholeness. The negative must be rebuked and replaced by renewing the mind-set. A person is free to choose life or death or to become detained on their spiritual journey. Try yoga and meditation along with prayer, which are an ancient art and science that is still as powerful and useful as it was centuries ago - this will enhance your spiritual path. As you seek to gain and give a spiritual offering, read these words by William Law (1686-1761):

> "But the spirit of prayer, the spirit of love, and the spirit of humility, or of any other virtue are only to be attained by the operation of the light and spirit of God, not outwardly teaching, but inwardly bringing forth a new-born spirit within us."

49

Summary

Becoming Transformed

"Don't be conformed to this world(earthy/human ways), but be ye transformed (remade, reborn, re-means to do over again) by the renewal of your mind (Spirit ways), so that (You) may prove what is the good and acceptable and perfect will of God, even the thing which is good and acceptable." (Romans 12:2)

Dearest Reader,

You should now have a clearer idea on "how to" develop a mystic consciousness. Learning from this book, yoga is an ancient old practice from over 4,000 years. It is an overall, healing practice. The physical, mental, emotional and spiritual of oneself will become integrated and united with their Higher Power by applying this practice into their life. This is apparent for traditional Christians, New Thought Christians, as well as non- Christians. Many busy professionals, performing artists, ministers and homemakers have found their quality of life is enhanced by taking time to meditate and practice yoga. Their minds become still and refreshed.

For many years, and during their darkest spiritual period of time, there have been those who have been curious and sought a "mystic consciousness." Several seekers did not understand their own souls' yearning. While seeking, they move here and there as "mystical travelers." Numerous souls had teachers, spiritual ministers, or role models who learned from the Universal God first hand. Thus, they are called "mystic" no matter what planet they lived on and from what period of time. Jesus, the Master teacher for most people, was a mystic himself. Devout followers of any religion desire a saintly kind of relationship with the Divine Creator of all things. Yet, their studies do not give them a clear blueprint. However, most of the spiritual religious seekers are looking for a deeper meaning for their life's purpose, which is almost mystical to them. As they detach from their worldly goods and emotions from this secular world, these faithful seekers live a simple and contemplative life. As a recap, they still feel unworthy to grace their Divine, similar to Saint Teresa's feelings over 600 hundred years ago. Saint Teresa of Avila was the teacher for the monks and the nuns. She taught her students about the sacred things of contemplative mental prayer life and entering their inner castle. As they enter their inner castle in prayer, meditation, humility, trust, faith in their Beloved and implementing their spiritual practice, they have all the tools the blueprint needs for purification of Divine union with their God. One must understand and know that mystic teachers faced their inner doubts daily, just like their followers, as noted by Saint John of the Cross, Saint Teresa's close companion, who gave her the insights and answers into her soul. She entered the "dark nights of the soul," just like anyone who is seeking a higher Union with their Beloved. Years went by and the Bishops could not answer her questions of why she felt so unworthy, numb, isolated and depressed. She called Saint John "the father of her soul." Now, you have answers to your soul's yearnings.

When one enters into solitude, silence and isolation, they may express it with art, poetry, music, prayer and meditation and dance. As they awaken into the light of their Universal God, the Spirit of God will purify and illuminate their paths. Then, there is still the "dark nights of the soul" one enters into, which is mostly unknown to the person. One must know and learn that if it is really depression, one must seek medical attention. Furthermore, if the darkness is still inside the soul, then it is a spiritual lesson that can only be lifted by the Universal God in due season. This too will pass. The "Gifts of depression" is a birthing time for a newness to evolve within one's soul, along with a time to die to the ego, false humility and pride. If one embraces this dark period with grace and ease, blessings come forth, such as writing, painting, songwriting, contemplation of speeches and research. One should welcome the darkness because light will come in due season, and the old self or life will no longer exist the way one knew it.

Seekers of a "mystic consciousness" have thought they must live in a convent, solitude or a monastery. This is not true for a higher spiritual walk in life. As one turns their mind, heart, spirit and soul to their center within, they will find everything needed. Saint Teresa taught the soul was like a mansion with many rooms. Each mystical spiritual seeker has a key that will open the door to become closer to the center of where the Beloved lived, if the key to understanding is used. The first key was prayer and meditation. A seeker will stay in that room until they understand how to apply the practice of mental prayers. The second key is developing a "spiritual practice," where every positive action done brings one so close to the Beloved. One will stay there until they apply this practice. Room three is the exemplary life; a seeker perfects their prayer life and maintains a high standard. A promise to marry is room four; so many seekers want to be married to someone in the flesh. Nevertheless, this is where the mystic life begins, with a soul mate, with the Beloved, a union. As an awareness of the Beloved increases, relapses are still possible, Saint Teresa taught. If one stays in this room long enough and masters the desire to marry, they will have a Comforter that will never leave - a flowing stream of comfort wrapped around ones' mind, spirit, soul and body without limits. Learning to surrender a personal Will to the Universal God is room five. The desire of God's Will is the seekers' desires. In the introduction of *Interior Castle* (Saint Teresa of Avila, p. 5), Saint Teresa tells us, "that one must infuse their thoughts with contemplation in order to grow in a Prayer of Union." The lover (seeker) and the Beloved (God) grow in love in room six. This is the stage that Evelyn Underhill wrote about. It affects the inside and the outside of the body through all types of sickness and discomforts. The Spiritual Marriage is a complete transformation in room seven, the Divine Call or Union.

 Many people have beaten themselves up spiritually for not understanding that they were going through the "dark nights of the soul." Have you? This information will shed light on your and another's spiritual pathway and guide their soul's spiritual journey. Thomas Moore writes, "If you give all your efforts to getting rid of your dark night, you may not learn its lessons or go through the important changes it can make for you. The dark nights of the soul are a period of transformation, which ends with a new discovery of self." (Moore p.16) This is the material I desire to share with those who are suffering and wish it to go away fast.

In Luke 4:23, it states, "Physician Heal Thyself." This is achieved by the yogi achieving and taking personal responsibility. One must give themselves permission to seek alternative and preventive measures for responsive healing. As one seeks medial counsel and trusts their inner guidance, they will do what is right for their body, mind and spirit.

One of the leading edge research and educational hospitals in the world, Mayo Clinic in Rochester, Minnesota, now refers and encourages the ancient practice of yoga and meditation to adult patients as well as children patients who have long-term illnesses. They are asked to invest just 20 minutes a day of meditation, yoga or Tai Chi. Researchers have found that participants gain a stronger immune system, lower blood pressure, increase flexibility, core stability, and balance to their conventional medical challenges. I would like to challenge you to try meditation, yoga or Tai Chi if you are not already, just for 20 minutes a day! Yoga, meditation and prayer are still as powerful and useful for gaining a spiritual awareness, just like it was centuries ago.

If Mother Teresa were here today with you, my dears, she would tell you this, from her book, Total Surrender:

"We should become empty from food, radio, or keeping busy. But this emptiness can only be filled by the "spiritual," by God. If we give time for God to enter this space, then our hunger can be more easily satisfied by just being with God in prayer. But it is hard thing to be prayerful in our society which feeds us with so many distractions."

Remember, Silence of the eyes seeking only goodness; Silence of the ears, following Gods promptings, to help the poor and watch our speech; Silence of the tongue, uplifting the Word of God and others;

Silence of the mind, being open to the truthfulness of God through prayer and contemplation. Only having pure thoughts about others and clear judgments. Silence of the heart, love God with everything within your cells, mind and heart. She says, "Our silence is a joyful and God-centered silence; it demands of us constant self-denial and plunges us into the deep silence of God where aloneness with god becomes a reality."

Namaste'
Carol S. Batey

After Thought ....

This book is filled with insights on meditation and other modalities on how to connect to that still, small voice. This voice is in each of us and is what connects us to our Creator. These teachings are meant to include everyone because the commonality of our oneness is universal. This is also applicable regardless of one's spiritual preference. All one needs is a willingness to apply these simple, yet profound practices that Carol sets forth. One cannot help but acquire what each of us so desperately seeks ... that "Mystic Consciousness."

Gene Skaggs, Author
A Beginner's Glossary to a Course in Miracles"

Bibliography

Anodea, Judith, and Selene Vega 1993
THE SEVENFOLD JOURNEY, Printed in the USA: 262

Batey, Carol S. 2009
POISE FOR THE RUNWAY OF YOUR LIFE, Bloomington, IN,
Author House

Beckwith, Michael Bernard 2008
SPIRITUAL LIBERATION: FULFILLING YOUR SOUL'S
POTENTIAL, New York, NY, Simon and Schuster

Browne, Sylvia 2008
MYSTICAL TRAVELER: HOW TO ADVANCE TO A HIGHER
LEVEL OF SPIRITUALITY, Carlsbad, CA, Hay House

Browne, Sylvia 2005
PHENOMENON: EVERYTHING YOU NEED TO KNOW
ABOUT THE PARANORMAL, London, England, Penguin Group

Colemon, Johnnie 2009
DAILY INSPIRATION, Miami Gardens, FL, Universal Foundation
for Better Living

Davis, Ph.D. Bruce 1990
MONASTERY WITHOUT WALLS, DAILY LIFE IN THE
SILENCE, Lincoln, NE, iUniverse.com

Feuerstein, Georg and Bodian Stephan 1993
LIVING YOGA, New York, Putnam Publishing Groups, 4-8,113,185

Fillmore, Charles 1959
    THE REVEALING WORD, Unity Village, MO, Unity House

Fillmore, Myrtle 2006
    HEALING LETTERS (UNITY CLASSIC LIBRARY), Unity
    Village, MO, Unity House

Flinders, Carol Lee 1993
    ENDURING GRACE, New York, NY, Harpers Collins

Foster, Richard J. and James Bryan Smith edited, 1990
    DEVOTIONAL CLASSICS, New York, NY, HarperCollins

Hennies, Ronald and Sonia Weiss 2004
    THE EVERYTHING PRAYER BOOK, Avon, MA, Adams Media

Hill, Napoleon et al. 2007
    THE PROSPERITY BIBLE, New York, NY, Jeremy P.
    Tacher/Penguin

Holmes, Ernest 1938
    THE SCIENCE OF MIND, New York, NY, Penguin Putman

Holy Bible 1979
    Nashville, TN, Thomas Nelson

Moore, Thomas 1994
    CARE OF THE SOUL, New York, NY, Harper Collins

Compiled by Lucinda Vardey 1997
    A SIMPLE PATH (Mother Teresa of Calcutta), Ballantine Books,
    New York, NY

Compiled by Jaya Chalika and Edward Le Joly 2000, THE JOY IN
    LOVING (Mother Teresa of Calcutta)., Penguin Group, New
    York, NY

Myss, Caroline 2001
    SACRED CONTRACTS: AWAKENING YOUR DIVINE
    POTENTIAL, New York, NY, Harmony Books

Pym, Jim 1999
    LISTENING TO THE LIGHT, London, England, SW IV, Random
    House

Saint John of the Cross 1959
    DARK NIGHT OF THE SOUL, New York, NY, Doubleday

Saint Teresa of Avila. Translation by E. Allison Peers 1946
    INTERIOR CASTLE. Mineola: Dover Publication

Translation by Mirabai Star 2007
    SAINT TERESA OF AVILA. Canada: Random House

Sinetar, Marsha 1996
    ORDINARY PEOPLE AS MONKS AND MYSTICS, Mahwah, NJ
    Paulist Press

Starr, Mirabai 2007
    TERESA OF AVILA: THE BOOK OF MY LIFE, Boston, MA
    New Seeds Book, Shambhala Publications, Inc.

Translation by Brother Angelo 1985
    TOTAL SURRENDER (Mother Teresa of Calcutta). Ann Arbor:
    Servant Publications, 1985

Trine, Ralph Waldo 1897
IN TUNE WITH THE INFINITE, New York, NY, Jeremy P.
Tacher/Penguin

Underhill, Evelyn 1993
MYSTICISM, Columbus, OH, Ariel Press

Zukav, Gary 1989
THE SEAT OF THE SOUL, New York, NY, Simon & Schuster

www.ingramcontent.com/pod-product-compliance
Lightning Source LLC
Chambersburg PA
CBHW031328290526
45784CB00014B/2434